Introduction

Herbs been around for 60,000 years. All modern medicine comes from herbs. Modern medicine is artificial form of the herbs. Modern medicine does more harm than good. Modern medicine has more chemicals that dissolve the purpose for the herb to work in modern medicine form. Herbs is the best solution to keep a body healthy strong and the only thing can heal the body naturally without side effects. Herbs heals every part of the body compare to modern medicine it only focuses one part of the body.

In this book, I will provide all the herbs that can help with different parts of the body. Then I will provide herbs that help heal your body from illness and diseases. After I will talk about the diets and drinks that are healthy for your diet and life style. Also, I will talk about vitamins you can take keep your overall health healthy and strong. This is a health book that give you the answers you need to live a natural lifestyle without harmful chemicals that will destroy and bandage the problem than cure it.

Table Content

Continue Table Contents

Brain Health

Brain is the most important organ in the body because it controls most of our body. Here are the herbs that can keep the brain healthy: (Make sure its organic form)

Turmeric

Centella asiatica

Bacopa

Ashwagandha

Asian Ginseng

Ginkgo biloba

Bacopa monnieri

Sage

Ginkgo

Lemon Balm

Lion's mane

Rhodiola rosea

Rosemary

Green Tea

Convolvulus pluricaulis

German chamomile

Hemp oil

Brain Health Continue

French lavender

Nutmeg

Gurana

Ginger

Cinnamon

Gaia

Licorice

Peppermint

Saffron

Heart Health

Heart is a special vessel of the body. We have to make sure our heart stays healthy and strong. Here are some herbs to help maintain heart health:(Make sure its organic form)

Garlic

Hawthorn

Cinnamon

Turmeric

Ginger

Asian Ginseng

Linden

Guggul

Reishi

Arjun Tree

Cayenne

Ginkgo

Green Tea

Hibiscus

Olive

Black seed oil

Heart Health Continue

Fenugreek

Red Sage

Coriander

Tulsi

Allium sativum

Aloe vera

Berberine

Nerve Health

Nerves are very important part of our body system because without our nerves we wouldn't be able to feel, muscles wouldn't be able to move and have no control on the major functions like digestive system. Here are herbs can help keep our nerves intact: (Make sure its organic form)

Passion Flower

Valerian

Lemon balm

Chamomile

Ashwagandha

Lavender

Matricaria chamomilla

Blue skullcap

Rhodiola rosea

Skullcap

Hemp oil

Continue of Nerve Health

Ginkgo biloba

American ginseng

Kava

Avena sativa

Bacopa

Basil

Catnip

Elaeagnus angustifolia

Melisa

Motherwort

Oatstraw

Ocimum sanctum

Passiflora incarnata

Circulatory Health

Circulatory is very important part of your health because it keeps our blood flowing and if your blood stop flowing properly then it causes health problems. Here are some herbs that can help with your circulatory system: (Make sure its organic form)

Ginger

Garlic

Ginkgo

Turmeric

Hawthorn

Cayenne Pepper

Centella asiatica

Olive

Bilberry

Chickweed

Chili

Citrus fruits

Green tea

Hawthorn berry

Bacopa

Continue Circulatory Health

Asian Ginseng

Hibiscus

Cinnamon

Grapeseed oil extract

Capsicum

Gingko biloba

Tincture

Horse chestnut

Allium

Astragalus

Berberine

Lung Health

Lungs is one of your valuable organs for your respiratory system. Even though we can live with one but it bests to protect both. Here are some herbs that help support lungs: (Make sure its organic form)

Licorice

Thyme

Mullein

Peppermint

Plantain

Eucalyptus

Ginger

Nettle

Elecampane

Horehound

Continue Lung Health

Astragalus

Blackseed oil

Oregano

Turmeric

Bayberry

Langwort

Marshmallow

Long Pepper

Vasaka

Anise

Garlic

Ginseng

OSHA

Parasite, Toxins and Detox Health

It's good to cleanse your body a least once or twice a month to keep the toxins, radicals and parasites out of your body.

Toxins and Detox (Make sure its organic form)

Cilantro

Dandelion

Milk Thistle

Red Clover

Turmeric

NAC (Augmented)

K2

Green Tea

Nattokinase

Monoatomic Gold (Ormus)

Parasites (Make sure its organic form)

Anise

Barberry

Berberine

Black walnut

Continue Detox, Toxins and Parasites

Clove oil

Goldthread

Goldenseal

Grapefruit seed oil

Propolis

Oregano oil

Oregano grape

Wormwood

Bone Health

Bone health is very important because our bones keep our body in shape. Weak bones cause many problems like extreme pain and arthritis. Here are some herbs that help with bone health:

(Make sure its organic form)

Red Sage

Red Clover

Horsetail

Thyme

Turmeric

Eyes Health

Eyes give us the sense to see and visual. The weakness of the eyes disturb our vision and it affect daily lives to do things. Here are some herbs that can help the eyes: (Make sure its organic form)

Gingko biloba

Bilberry

Eyebright

Turmeric

Fennel

Green tea

Grapeseed

Continue to Eye Health

Saffron

Basil

Calendula

German chamomile

Coleus

Goldenseal

Passion flower

Bilberries

Buddleia flower buds

Buddleja officinalis

Tea plant

Cannabis

Chrysanthemum flower

Milk thistle

Wolfberries

Letein

Bentonite clay

Skin, Hair and Nails Health

Skin, Hair and Nails are very important part of your health. When these three things are healthy then your body is healthy and if these are unhealthy then it indicates there is something wrong with your health. Here are some herbs can maintain good health for nails, hair and skin:

(Make sure its organic form)

Burdock

Nettles

Centella asiatica

Horsetail

Rosemary

Alfalfa

Ashwagandha

Calendula

German Chamomile

Ginkgo

Green tea

Lavender

Peppermint

Triphala

Turmeric

Aloe vera

Saw Palmetto

Argan oil

Coconut oil

Shea Butter

Hemp oil

Tea tree oil

Saw Palmetto

Avocado oil

Olive oil

Emotional and Mental Health

Emotional and Mental health is very important because when these two aren't right it disturb the rest of your body and you aren't functionally right. Here are some herbs that can help with that:

(Make sure its organic form)

Perforate St. John-wort

German chamomile

Passion flower

Lemon balm

Ashwagandha

Lavender

Valerian

Saffron

English lavender

Oat

Rhodiola

Rhodiola rosea

Continue Emotional and Mental Health

Persian Silk tree

Cannabis sativa

Ginkgo

References

Rose

Rosemary

Skullcap

Kava

Withania somnifera

Ginseng

Linden

Piper methysticum

Digestive Health

Every disease starts from the gut. So, if our gut isn't good then diseases start to rise and start issues from cancer to diabetes. It always good to maintain our overall gut health. Here are some herbs that can help and support the digestive system: (Make sure its organic form)

Turmeric

Cardamom seed

Milk thistle seed

Dandelion root

Gentian root

Ginger root

Slippery elm

Peppermint

Oregano

Aloe vera

Black pepper

Sugar Health (Pancreas and Insulin)

Everyone wants a functional insulin that regulate our blood sugar. When blood sugar isn't healthy then it causes problems like diabetes, pancreas cancer and more. Here are some herbs that help with insulin: (Make sure its organic form)

Fenugreek

Ginger

Tumeric

Bitter melon

Gymnema

Berberine

Curry tree

Gingko

Holy basil

Sage

Cayenne

Oregano

Rosemary

Aloe vera

Cinnamon

Ginseng

Trigonella foenum graecum

Momordica charantica

Opuntia Streptacantha

Milk Thistle

Immune Health

Immune system is very important to help fight infections, viruses and bacteria. Our immune system has to be strong in order to fight these antigens. If our immune system is weak, we become sick and ill. Here are some herbs can help build up your immune system: (Make sure its organic form)

Seamoss

Blackseed oil

Grapeseed oil

NAC

Black Elderberry

Echinacea

Andrographis

Astragalus

Calendula

Cat's claw

Goldenseal

Lomatium

Myrrh

Olive

Oregano

Propolis

Reishi

Respiratory Health

Already talk about lung health. Respiratory health as a whole is very important. A lot illness attacks this system when we sick so it best to protect this system as much as possible. Here some herbs that help support the respiratory system: (Make sure its organic form)

Thyme

Licorice

Plantain

Ginger

Mullein

Nettle

Peppermint

Elecampane

Marshmallow

Eucalyptus

Oregano

Continue Respiratory Health

Anise

Astragalus

Blackseed oil

Goldenseal

Horsehead

Long Pepper

Vasaka

Marshmallow

Bayberry

Turmeric

Echinacea

Tulsi

Energy Health

Its very important to have sufficient amount of energy throughout the day, If not we are very tire, fatigue, emotional, depress and don't feel like doing anything. Here are some herbs can help with energy boost: (Make sure its organic form)

Asian Ginseng

Ashwagandha

Rhodiola rosea

Maca

Schisandra

Eleuthero

Bacopa

Cordyceps

Ginkgo

Green tea

Tulsi

Peppermint

Continue Energy Health

Centella asiatica

Gurana

Astragalus Propinquus

Sage

Gaia

Cola

Matcha

Shilajit

Yerba mate

Cayenne

Reproductive Health

Reproductive system is very important because it controls the function of our hormones and our sexual abilities. Here are some herbs that help maintain our reproductive system: (Make sure its organic form)

Chaste tree

Red clover

Ashwagandha

Maca

Black cohosh

Dong quai

Saw Palmetto

Cramp bark

Damiana

Evening Primrose Oil

False unicorn

Continue Reproductive Health

Licorice

Motherwort

Red raspberry

Shatavari

Tribulus

Wild yam

Agnus Castus

Ptychopetalum

Ricinus

German chamomile

Cinnamon

Liver and Kidney Health

The same as digestive system, we have to keep our liver and kidney health in order because they keep our system flush out from toxins and radicals. Here are some herbs that can support and maintain liver and kidney health: (Make sure its organic form)

Turmeric

Milk Thistle

Dandelion

Liquorice

Ginger

Artichoke

Selenium

Green tea

Asian Ginseng

Astragalus Propinquus

Garlic

Parsley

Chanca Piedra

Triphala

Aloe vera

Ear Health

Ear health is very important because it connected with the immune system and the brain system. It always good makes sure to take probiotics and herbs to help keep this function intact. Never good to have an earache or an infection. Here some herbs that help support the ears: (Make sure its organic form)

Basil

Oregano

Tumeric

Dill

Oral & Teeth Health

Oral and Teeth Health is very important because it cause gum diseases and affect the heart if isn't taken care of probably. Here some herbs that help oral and teeth: (Make sure its organic form)

Peppermint

Basil

Clove

Turmeric

Myrrh

Echinacea

Sage

Bloodroot

Eucalyptus

Garlic

Goldenseal

Rosemary

Thyme

Neem

Cinnamon

Green tea

Cancer

Cancer unalive millions of people every year. If people live their lives with a proper diet, liquids, cleaning the body and take herbs can help reduce this disease. Here are some herbs that can support, minimize and heal: (Make sure its organic form)

Tumeric

Ginger

Cayenne Pepper

Garlic

Echinacea

Gingko

Ginseng

Omega 3

Vitamin D

Probiotics

Selenium

Zinc

Vitamin E

Diabetes

Half the population is diagnosis with diabetes, the proper diet, exercise, drinks and environment can help this problem and avoid all together. Here are some herbs can help heal and support diabetes: (Make sure its organic form)

Gymnema sylvestre

Tumeric

Berberine

Ocimum basilicum

Gingko Phyllanthus amarus

Bitter melon

Oregano

Allium

Cayenne

Cinnamomum

Barbary Fig

Fenugreek

Pterocarpus marsupium

Heart Diseases

Heart diseases are very concerning in our country. Many people are unalive every day from some form of heart disease. If people lead healthy life style than they can avoid these issues. Here are some herbs that help support heart diseases: (Make sure its organic form)

Garlic

Asian Ginseng

Ginger

Hawthorn

Tumeric

Green tea

Gingko

Hibiscus

Red sage

Cinnamon

Cayenne

Corlander

Olive leaf

Blood Health (High Blood Pressure)

Blood pressure correlates with heart disease. So, when blood pressure is high it can cause a stroke, heart attack and diabetes. If people practice healthy diet and exercise you can avoid this health problem. (Make sure its organic form)

Cinnamon

Garlic

Basil

Parsley

Celery seeds

Thyme

Ginger

Chinese cat's claws

Bacopa monnieri

Diets and Drinks

Its very important to live a healthy life style to avoid illness and diseases. So, you or your family have to pick a diet and drinks that will help your family thrive. Let's talk about the diets and the drinks.

Diets

Vegan is a diet that focus on vegetables and fruits. Most people eat raw and others will cook food time and time again. They don't eat no dairy products. They avoid carbs as much as they can and they depend on herbs. No meat at all.

Vegetarian is a diet that focus on vegetables, fruits, dairy products and carbs. They eat raw and cook food. They use herbs occasionally. They eat plant base meat products. No real meat.

Pescatarian is a diet that focus on vegetables, fruits, dairy products, carbs and seafood. They eat raw and cook food. They use herbs if necessary. They eat seafood and plant base products. No chicken or red meat.

Pollartian is a diet that focus on vegetables, fruits, dairy products, carbs, and chicken. They eat raw and cook food. They don't really depend on herbs. They eat chicken and sometimes plant base products. No seafood or red meat.

Pesci-Pollartian is a diet that focus on vegetables, fruits, diary products, carbs, chicken and seafood. They eat cook food mostly and some raw food. Herbs isn't really necessary form them. They eat chicken, seafood and some plant base. No red meat.

After these diets, you eat red meat in your diet then you putting your health more of risk compare to having white meat in your diet or no meat at all.

Drinks

The best H20 to drink is alkaline, spring and distill water. Purified water has to much process and chemicals that are added and harmful to health.

H30 is water that comes from coconuts, herbs and fruits. It best to intake from the food we eat vs. drinking the water unless you know where it comes from.

Organic juice is the best juice to drink if you like juice. Don't drink to much and for children mix it with water.

Coconut Milk, Oat Milk and Almond milk is the best milk drink. If you don't like these then you can drink goat milk compare to cow milk.

Beside these four drinks are the best liquids you can drink and it best to avoid sugary drinks like soda, tea, Gatorade and etc.

Superfood

These are herbs and spices that are superfood for your overall diet. (Make sure its organic form)

Cardamom

Carob

Chocolate – Dark and organic

Cinnamon

Coffee – Organic

Cranberries

Currant

Fennel

Garlic

Ginger

Parsley

Peppercorn

Rosemary

Sage

Tea

Turmeric

Seamoss

Vitamins

We have vitamins that we have to intake to maintain overall health. Here the list vitamins: (Make sure its organic form)

K2

D3

Vitamin C

Vitamin B12

Vitamin B complex

Magnesium

Potassium

Calcium

Zinc

Omega 3

Copper

Selenium

Iron

Iodine

Sodium

Vitamin A and E (needed for some)

Final Words

Herbs been here for us to use. We aren't suppose to depend on modern medicine. We suppose to depend on the herbs and ourselves. We not suppose to put trust in the doctors and the system. We can take care ourselves and live a long time. Just practice a healthy lifestyle put vegetables and fruits first, add herbs and spices, drink healthy products, exercise and live stress free. Always make sure the herbs, vegetables, fruits and drinks are in their purist form, non-gmo and organic. Your life depends on you and not the world.

Other Books

My Life Lessons Journey by Sharika Kkkyha

Remove Self from Society by Sharika Flores

The Transition from Public School to Homeschool by Rica Kanesha K.F.

Homeschool Curriculum books coming soon

Books in audio form coming soon (will be available on Amazon, Audible and iTunes)

Made in the USA
Columbia, SC
06 March 2025

54712849R00024